The Alkaline Diet Solution

How to Lose Weight Faster and Live
Healthier with a PH Balanced Diet

J.C. Collins

**Limits of Liability, Disclaimer of Warranties & Terms of
Use**
This book is a general educational health-related information
product. As an express condition to reading this book, you
understand and agree to following terms. The information and
advice contained in this book are not intended as a substitute for
consulting with a healthcare professional.

The publisher and authors are not responsible for any adverse
effects or consequences resulting from the use of any of the
suggestions, or procedures discussed in this book. While all
attempts have been made to verify information provided in this
book, the author and publisher assume no responsibility for
errors, omissions, or contrary interpretation of the subject
matter herein. All matters pertaining to your physical health
should be supervised by a health care professional

ISBN-10: 1501050540
ISBN-13: 978-1501050541

DEDICATION

This book is dedicated to those in search of an effective way to lose weight and live a healthier lifestyle through The Alkaline Diet.

CONTENTS

INTRODUCTION

There many different dieting programs advertised to the public today and choosing one that is safe and effective is quite confusing. Trying to identify the flaws from all these diet programs can be complicated. Meanwhile, learning more about the acid alkaline system will give you a better understanding as to why it is worth a try.

Alkaline dieting is synonymous to healthy eating. Unlike many crash diet programs that promote starvation or the use of dieting pills, the alkaline diet program promotes awareness in eating the right kinds of food that sustain the nutritional needs of our body. Eating correctly is accompanied by following an exercise routine that suits your body condition and staying away from unhealthy habits like smoking and excessive drinking.

It's not about being able to lose weight quickly and then going back to old, unhealthy eating habits afterwards. It isn't a temporary loss of unwanted pounds that you'll soon gain back only a few months after you stopped the diet. In fact, it's not just about achieving the ideal body weight. The alkaline system is all about practicing healthy eating and living a more satisfying life.

CHAPTER 1 – WHAT IS THE ALKALINE DIET?

The alkaline diet is composed of foods that prevent the increase of acid levels in the body. It keeps the pH balance at normal range and maintains the normal function of other body fluids. This diet is also responsible in preventing or treating certain diseases in bladder and bloodstreams.

The traditional alkaline diet is one that is devoid of poultry, cheese and meat. This way, the urine environment could be altered so as to avoid the growth of kidney stones and prevent urinary tract infections.

The alkaline diet has also been used by some medicine practitioners to treat or prevent low energy levels, heart disease, and cancer among other diseases.

Later on, the diet was popularized by many fitness experts as an effective diet for weight loss. With its ability to help increase the energy levels of the body, one can maximize the body's capacity in exercise and other activities that help burn unwanted fats.

Alkaline Diet Composition

According to the traditional theory of this diet, the alkaline ash is produced by vegetables and fruits, except prunes, plum, and blueberries. In some hypothesis performed by student doctors, it was found that the alkaline ash elements can decrease the risk of osteoporosis. The National Academy of Sciences made further research and confirmed the said hypothesis.

Food Consumption

In alkaline diet, you can eat most vegetables, tofu and soybeans, some nuts, legumes, and seeds. On the other hand, meat, eggs, dairy, most grains, processed foods like packaged snacks, canned goods and convenience foods are not allowed; these foods fall under the category of 'acid-promoting foods'. Most alkaline diet experts are also prohibiting the intake of alcohol and caffeine.

Alkaline diet works completely for vegetarians as well as for vegans, since dairy is off-limits. The diet restricts the consumption of wheat, but in order to avoid gluten, one must carefully examine all food labels because gluten is not only present in wheat. Aside from wheat, the diet also prohibits the intake of allergy-triggering foods such as fish, shellfish, walnuts, peanuts, and milk. For this cause, the diet is also perfect for people who are trying to avoid sugar.

With all these restrictions, some people find the diet very hard to keep. Aside from all the foods that must be avoided, it may also take a while before you get used to preparing an alkaline diet meal. The looks may not be as interesting as the ones you have been used to eating. Nonetheless, due to the many benefits it offers, more and more people, including some famous personalities and Hollywood actors are on it.

J.C. Collins

CHAPTER 2 – ALKALINE DIET: ACHIEVE REAL WEIGHT LOSS

Gareth Edwards, an expert on Alkaline Diet for weight loss, had shared many ways on how to stay healthy and achieve permanent results just through following the said diet.

Some people who went on this diet said they gained instead of lose weight but Edwards said that it isn't the case with his clients. Interestingly, many of his clients come to him not because their main goal is to lose weight but because they want to rid of the accompanying health problems of having excess fats.

Edwards prompted that when a person wants to lose weight, he actually wants to become healthier in reality. This is the reason why he worked to look for ways that can boost up the effects of alkaline diet to everyone who wants to lose weight in no time.

Many clients of Edward have experimented following alkaline diet alongside with an excellent hydration and exercise program. But after a few weeks, nothing has changed and problems in weight and health persist. Edwards pointed out that this is because depriving oneself with foods while embarking on hard core exercises won't be easy at first. Even with alkaline diet, people will be tempted to overeat to fill in the loss of energy. But with the proper combination of meals included in alkaline diet, one can achieve his ultimate goal of losing weight while keeping his body strong through daily exercise.

The Importance of Greens

The common thing that you can hear from people who are already keeping alkaline diet is that they successfully lose weight when they began eating lots of foods coming from green plants. Included in the list are kale, chard, watercress, parsley, spinach, wheatgrass, cucumbers, and some green leaves.

These plant foods have properties that deal with weight gaining problems. First, they are all low in sugar, and the number one requirement in any weight loss program is to reduce the amount of sugar intake. They are also high in nutrients and vitamins that are responsible for revitalizing and energizing the body.

Moreover, when eaten raw, they produce high levels of electrons and an alkalizing negative charge. This property encourages the flow of energy throughout your body.
These foods also contain high amounts of magnesium, which is essential to make the heart pump as well as to help eliminate body waste. They are also filled with chlorophyll, which helps build healthy red blood cells that are important to the process of weight loss.

High levels of fiber can also be found in these healthy foods. Fiber is one of the major helpful factors in eliminating body waste, keeping it free from fats as well as toxins and many harmful elements inside the body.

J.C. Collins

CHAPTER 3 – ESSENTIAL ALKALINE DIET BEVERAGES

The fastest way to make effective any kind of weight loss program is by drinking lots of water. The body responds easier to detoxification when it is properly hydrated. Next to oxygen, water is considered to be a critical element in facilitating and maintaining the chemistry of the body.

The general advice for most adults is to drink at least 8 glasses of water. You may get the proper amount of water that your body needs by finding your weight and dividing it into two. For example, if you weigh 160 lbs, divide 160 into two and you will get 80, which means you need to consume at least 80 oz. of water per day.

The body activity and environment must also be considered in order to know the right amount of water needed. If you are an active person, like an athlete, or if you live in a dry place, then you needed more water. Water poses no danger to the body so the more water you drink, the better.

Pure water is important to match with your alkaline diet. If your water system is not safe, it is highly recommended to get an excellent water filtration system of your own. It may mean additional expense on your account, but it would ensure that you will safely get the pure water that you need as you go on an alkaline diet.

If you are going to buy bottled drinking water, make sure to get the alkaline type. You may also choose to alkalize your own water by using alkalizing agents such as Prime pH. Alkalizing the water adds oxygen to the water and it also neutralizes its acid content.

Avoid Acidic Drinks: Tea, Coffee, Soda, etc.

You need to avoid all acidic drinks in general.

The body works its way in maintaining its pH balance. In order to keep the alkalinity in balance, it must always range between 7.36 – 7.37. When you drink more acidic beverages, you are basically breaking this balance. Imbalanced pH level will result to death.

In order to save the body, the inner system will work to keep the acids away and put them somewhere else. These acids are eventually placed in fat cells, where it can do no immediate harm but would slowly poison your body, making you fat and more prone to different kinds of diseases.

So while you enjoy drinking any kind of acidic beverages, your body is already filling up your fat cells with poisonous acids. And the more acid you take, the more you get fat and unhealthy.

Here is a simple equation of the acid content of some drinks:

Water = Neutral
Tea = 600 to 800 times more acidic
Coffee = 700 to 1,000 times more acidic
Soda = 50,000 times more acidic
What does that shows?

If you really want to lose weight, and if you really want to follow alkaline diet effectively, then you must give up all your cravings for acidic beverages and liquids such as coffee, soda, tea (except herbal), beer, Gatorade, Red Bull, hard liquor, malted beverages and vinegar. Replace all of these with pure drinking water, and losing weight will become so easy.

Alkaline Beverages

Immune Booster Alkaline Juice
It is a mixture of tomatoes, cucumber and celery. This juice is filled with plenty of alkalinity, nutrients, and vitamins to prevent you from feeling less energized during the winter season.

Tomatoes are rich in lycopene and are known for being rich in antioxidants. Cucumbers, on the other hand, contain plenty of phytonutrients and lignans that help prevent the development of many diseases. Lastly, celery offers anti-inflammatory benefits and has heaps of flavonoids, Vitamin C and other anti-oxidants.

Ingredients:
1 celery stalk,
2 tomatoes,
½ cucumber,
2 cloves of garlic,

juice of 1 lemon

Use a juicer to extract the juice from all ingredients, including the cloves of garlic. Remember to wash the juicer right after usage to immediately remove the remains of garlic. Otherwise, all the juice that you will make for the next seven days will have a hint of garlic in them.

Alkaline Refresher Juice
This juice produces the detoxifying, alkalizing, and antioxidant benefits from grapefruits; it provides the sweetness and delicious taste of carrots; it brings out the refreshing taste of celery; and it gives the drinker the zing of a strong ginger.

Ingredients:
2 grapefruits,
2 stalks of celery,
1 carrot, an inch of ginger,
and 250 ml of alkaline water.
This amount makes 2 servings.

Wash all the ingredients thoroughly then peel the ginger and grapefruit. Put everything in the juicer and juice them together. Serve with or without ice.

Alkaline Margarita
Here's an excellent alcohol alternative for you that you can drink on your own or when there is a special occasion and you simply want to have a toast. This is a great way of indulging yourself with a great tasting beverage without blowing off your diet.

Ingredients: Makes two servings
One lemon,
two limes,
four sticks of celery,

one cucumber,
one inch of root ginger,
and Himalayan salt (optional).

Instructions:

Peel the lime and lemon. To produce the juice, you may use a juicer or simply slice them into halves and squeeze each with your bare hands. Set the juice aside.

Peel the ginger and juice it.

Juice the remaining ingredients and mix them all together afterwards. Add as much ginger as you like; it will add a little spice on your refreshing drink. Sprinkle a desired amount of Himalayan salt to complete the taste of this drink.

J.C. Collins

CHAPTER 4- ESSENTIAL ALKALINE DIET FOODS

The concept that holds true for acidic beverages applies the same for poisonous foods. Foods that can poison the body include preservatives, synthetic additives, and coloring.

The body is not designed to digest these chemicals so it does either of the following:

1. Eliminate the chemicals;
2. Neutralize them;
3. Store them away in a place where they can immediately damage the body.

If the body is not properly hydrated, then there's no assurance that it can eliminate these chemicals. So the body will be left with the options number 2 and 3. In the previous chapter, it has already been discussed where the poisons are stored away, so let's take a closer look at number 2.

In order to neutralize acids, the body system will create

and pull alkaline buffers from any place it can, then:
It will create cholesterol so as to neutralize acids, which is the main reason why many people suffer from high cholesterol levels.

- It will bleach the iron from red blood cells, which is how anemia starts to develop.
- It will pull calcium from bones, which is the main cause of osteoporosis.
- It will steal potassium from muscle tissues, which causes muscle spasms.
- It will pull magnesium, zinc, and many other elements from different parts of the body.

All of these will create additional health problems to the body. Moreover, the entire process will force the body to work full time, putting to waste all the energy you've worked on in order to produce neutralizing toxins. This energy could have been used more effectively in keeping the body active and help lose weight.

From now on, take time in reading the food labels. It will not only save your from poisoning yourself but you will also be able to save more money from the bills you will have to pay when you get sick.

Avoid Artificial Sweeteners

Many people who are trying to lose weight rely on artificial sweeteners in order to cut calories. These sweeteners include saccharin, NutraSweet, sucralose, and aspartame. Consuming these sweeteners would be like trying to kill yourself.

Sweeteners are far worse than alcohol, preservatives and acids. They pose problems on acid elimination process, as well as affect many other parts of the body in serious ways.

In countless studies, NutraSweet, which was the commercial name for Aspartame, was linked to serious damage in nervous system and cause neurological problems. Saccharin, on the other hand, contains a chemical that can cause cancer though most manufacturers would tell you that it can't happen to you. Would you risk it?

The bottom line is that by drinking or eating any artificial sweeteners, you are literally throwing off your efforts in losing weight. Additionally, consuming sweeteners would be an act of destroying one's body in ways that may no longer be repairable.

Sugar Substitute

Stevia is a sweetener that comes from the leaves of a plant of the same name. It is an excellent sugar substitute and a healthier one compared to artificial sweeteners. It is highly recommended by doctors and has been generally recognized as safe to be used as food additives. So if you are planning to set up an alkaline meal of your own, use Stevia to sweeten your food.

Quick Snack

Fighting constant cravings is the major problem when trying to lose weight. Following the alkaline diet requires much dedication that it would be a whole lot harder to take than any other diet plans.

However, alkaline diet helps reduce cravings over time. It works naturally that somehow, you will no longer feel like you are restricting yourself from foods that you have been used to eating for a long time.

When dealing with cravings, one must understand how the

body works with regards to food. Most people can't recognize the difference between hunger and thirst signal. When they feel hydrated, they turn to food to satisfy their stomach. On the other hand, this can't be a big issue when you are following the earlier advice on keeping the body properly hydrated by drinking lots of water every day.

The first step in dealing with craving is to recognize the source - is it from thirst or from hunger? When you feel hungry, drink two glasses of water and wait for a minute or two. If you find yourself still craving for something, then eat something that is good for you. The trick here is to move your jaw into action. The safest and most effective trick is by chewing some soaked nuts and raw, cut vegetables. These foods have the bigger crunch and would require you to chew longer while taking a large part in your stomach.

When you go out to the grocery, choose cut vegetables that are fresh. Better yet, find a wholesale club or a farmer's market where you can purchase organic foods at affordable prices. You may also opt to look for a variety of hummus to dip your cut vegetables in for added taste.

Among many nuts, the best ones to soak are hazelnuts, walnuts and almonds. Among the three, almonds taste the best, fill up your stomach the better and are the most alkalizing.

Before soaking the almonds, rinse them first in cold water. As you rinse, rub them carefully, then put them in a bottle. Fill the container with water. You have to ensure that there is enough water to cover all the almonds as they grew fuller. Store the container in a refrigerator overnight. The next morning, take the almonds from the water and dry them with a paper towel. The almonds are now ready to eat. To store the remains, put them in an airtight container and keep them refrigerated. The soaked fresh almonds can last for about 5 to 7 days.

The other nuts are soaked in the same way, but they only need about 4 to six hours of soaking.

Tip: Bring your soaked nuts and cut vegetables with you anywhere you go. When you feel like eating a snack, take the nuts instead of buying junk foods. You may keep them in a Ziploc bag for convenience.

Delicious Alkaline Diet Meals

Alkaline Wrap-less Wraps
Wraps are one of the favorites among delicious snacks. Replace those bread wraps with something more alkaline, and you'll then have a healthier meal that will also help you stay fit.

Ingredients: Good for 2 servings
2 ripe avocadoes,
2 ripe tomatoes,
6 large lettuce leaves,
½ fresh chili,
½ onion (medium),
juice of 1 organic lemon,
and 1 pinch of Himalayan crystal salt or crystal sea salt.

Instructions:
Mash the avocadoes with a fork in a bowl. Set it aside then chop the red onions, tomatoes, parsley and coriander into small pieces. You may also chop the chili if you want to. Then sprinkle the salt and squeeze the lemon's juice over the mashed avocado and mix it together with all the other chopped stuff. It would produce something like salsa, but is more alkaline and healthy with its avocado content. Set aside.

Now, take the lettuce leaves. Wash them immensely and pat them dry.

Distribute the mixture among the leaves. Wrap each leaf and secure them with a cocktail stick.

Spinach Tofu Burgers

It's great to find a way to make a healthy burger. This Spinach Tofu Burger is gluten-free and is deliciously healthy for the body.

Ingredients:
15 ounces of firm tofu,
16 ounces of frozen organic spinach (thawed),
¾ cup of gluten-free rolled oats,
1 medium onion,
3 to 4 cloves of minced garlic,
¼ cup of LSA mix,
1 tablespoon of paprika,
1 teaspoon of cumin,
¼ cup of coconut oil,
and salt and pepper for added taste.
Optional Addition: A dash of Liquid Amino

Instructions:
Disintegrate the tofu then mix all the other ingredients in a bowl. Leave the mixture for a few minutes to allow the oats to absorb some liquid from spinach.

If the mixture is not wet enough to stick together, you may add a little water. Also add the liquid amino if desired.
Mold patties with your bare hands and then fry them in coconut oil. Cook each side for about 6 to 10 minutes, turning each patty carefully. Serve it afterwards with a nice salad.

Creamy Brussels

Brussels is a nutritious cruciferous. It has chemicals that prevent cancer. This creamy meal boosts the repair of damaged cells and blocks the growth of cancer cells.

Ingredients: Good for 1 serving only
Five to ten Brussels sliced into halves,
1 to 2 tablespoon of tahini,
1 tablespoon of coconut oil,
1 to 2 teaspoons of Bragg,
and 1 to 2 tablespoons of toasted sesame seeds.

Instructions:
Steam all Brussels within 8 to 10 minutes or until they start softening, but don't allow them to go mushy or lose their color. Afterwards, drain the water off. Place it into a pan, add oil and sauté until it gets golden brown. While the Brussels cook, take the tahini and mix it with Bragg in a bowl. Add a little water if the mixture got really thick.

Once the Brussels are cooked, turn off the stove and add the tahini and Bragg mixture. Mix it all together until all Brussels are coated. This should not produce a soupy mixture. If it becomes a little watery, turn the stove back on and cook until it dries a bit and thickens up.

When all the sprouts are already coated, place them on a plate or a bowl. Sprinkle the sesame seeds generously over the Brussels.

Avocado and Chickpea Mash

Avocado is considered to be one of the tastiest alkaline foods. Combine it with chickpeas and it would taste even better! Chickpeas are rich in fiber and protein, which makes it a perfect meal for people who are trying to lose weight.

Ingredients:
1 can of chickpeas
1 ripe avocado
Crackled black pepper and Himalayan salt
Flax Oil
Cumin
Optional: Choose an herb of your choice – parsley, basil, or coriander

Instructions:
In a medium sized bowl, mix together the drained chickpeas, sliced avocado, salt and pepper. Squeeze a pinch of cumin and sprinkle the herb of your choice over the mixture. Mix it again.

Put aside some of the whole chickpeas then mix all the ingredients again with the use of a large fork or a potato musher. Put back all the chickpeas to the mixture.

Drizzle some oil flax over and sprinkle paprika if desired. Serve it as you please.

This recipe is also perfect for salad and vegetable wraps.

CHAPTER 5 – NOURISHING ALKALINE SMOOTHIES

Smoothies are perfect on hot summer days. Fortunately there are perfect alkaline smoothies that can offer you coolness not only in summer days but in any day you like.

1.   Chocolate Smoothie

This smoothie is a combination of healthy fruits and vegetables. It produces a chocolate flavor and offers extra energy to help you get through a busy day.

Ingredients:
2 handfuls of spinach,
½ ripe avocado,
200 ml of almond milk,
200 ml of coconut milk,
3 teaspoon of coconut oil,
3 tablespoon of coconut yogurt
(or non-dairy yogurt, whichever you prefer),
3 tablespoon of raw cacao,

25 grams of soaked cashew,
50 grams of soaked almonds,
1 tablespoon of Maca powder (optional),
1 tablespoon of chia seeds,
and 1 tablespoon of sesame seeds.

Start preparing this smoothie by soaking the almonds and cashew. The perfect soaking time for nuts are discussed in chapter 4, but if you are in a hurry, soak the almonds and cashew for at least 20 minutes. Then, blend together the spinach, avocado and other liquids to produce a smooth paste. Once you have the paste, add the soaked nuts, the seeds and the yogurt. Blend them together within 10 seconds then add the maca and cacao. Lastly, before finishing the blend, add the oil.

Note: Maca has a strong taste. You may include or exclude it from the recipe. On the other hand, you may experiment putting a small amount and gradually increasing the amount until you find the exact taste that will meet your taste.

Nutritional Value:
Cacao provides antioxidant benefits, cellular support (that is required for the production of energy), energy producing minerals, and heart health benefits.

Maca is a nutritionally dense food that is filled with high amounts of vitamins, minerals, enzymes, and essential amino acids. It's not only beneficial for weight loss but is also excellent for hormonal balance, as a mood booster, and for skin protection.

2.   Grapefruit and Basic Greens Smoothie

This smoothie doesn't only provide high amounts of vitamin C but it is also delicious. Vitamin C, produced by

Grapefruit, helps in keeping the cardiovascular system healthy.

Ingredients:
1 avocado,
2 grapefruits (peeled and deseeded),
2 cups of fresh young spinach or other leafy greens,
1 pinch of stevia, and 4 ounces of water.
Mix everything, blend them together and you're good to go. This will make 2 servings.

3. Anti-Inflammatory Smoothie

This simple recipe can help prevent any kind of inflammation that might trigger when you start following the alkaline diet. According to many studies, turmeric and ginger are found to be more effective in fighting inflammation than prescription drugs.

Ingredients: Good for 2 servings
1 inch of grated fresh turmeric,
1 inch of grated ginger,
a handful of young spinach,
a handful of watercress,
1 small soft avocado,
1 cup of coconut or filtered water,
½ capsicum,
a handful of coriander or flat leaf parsley,
a big pinch of cayenne, and a pinch of salt.

Instructions:
Grate the turmeric and the ginger with a blender and mix the avocado and coconut water. Blend them together to produce a base. Then add all the remaining ingredients and blend them until the mixture becomes smooth.

4.　　Alkaline Antioxidant Green Smoothie

This smoothie is full of greens that are rich in anti-oxidants. Anti-oxidants help remove fat and cholesterol in the body, which can greatly help in keeping your body fit and healthy.

Ingredients:
a handful of spinach,
a handful of kale,
a handful of lettuce,
2 broccoli heads,
1 avocado,
1 tomato,
1 cucumber,
½ lemon,
½ clove of garlic,
and small amount of water according to your desired texture.

Instructions:
All you need to do is blend all the ingredients together. To form a mushy paste, you can start by blending lemon juice, cucumber and avocado then add the remaining ingredients afterwards.

Note: If you are just starting your alkaline diet and you find this smoothie to be too much crowded with vegetable taste, you may add any fruit of your choice to sweeten it up a bit. You can also put some capsicum for added sweetness.

5.　　Morning Smoothie

This smoothie is perfect to help you get started in the morning. You may drink it before and after your morning warm-up and exercise.

Ingredients:
Half cucumber
five sticks of celery
1/8 of cabbage
four handfuls of spinach or three kales
and juice of half a lemon

Mix all the ingredients and blend them together. Add some olive oil for added taste if you like.

J.C. Collins

CHAPTER 6 – HOW TO MAKE IT ALL WORK

A person who is used to eating anything he likes may find the alkaline diet very hard to follow. It's not easy to adhere in a diet where you will be restricted with almost everything that you have been eating all your life.

Here are some tips that you can follow through as you start following the alkaline diet:

1. Understand its benefits.

Alkaline diet offers a lot of benefits, as was discussed in the first chapter of this book. Keep these benefits in your mind to make it easier for you to turn your back when temptation arises.

2. Engage yourself in physical activities.

Join a sports club or a gym class in your community. Start your day with at least 15 minutes of cardiovascular exercise. If you prefer staying at home, buy aerobics CDs and exercise on your own.

With alkaline diet, you will feel more energized. That means you will have plenty of energy that you need to use on any kind of physical activity that you choose. By engaging yourself in exercises, you will be able to burn more calories and lose more fats in no time.

3. Mark your progress.

Keep a track on the progress of your alkaline diet. Mark the date of your start so you can see your accomplishment. This is one way of motivating yourself in keeping forward.

4. Tell a friend.

Share your goal with your spouse or friends. If they know about your diet plans, then it will be easier for you to continue socializing with them. Nowadays, people are becoming more aware of the great need for health awareness. Once your friends discover what you are up to, they might also want to join you and you will then have a group of people to start this diet with. Socializing with people who are pursuing the same alkaline diet will not only enrich the friendship bond, but will also help you keep the diet easier.

5. Consistency and Commitment

The main secret to success is to be committed and to be consistent with your plan. The odds may be hard at first but you will find it easier as you go on. Just continue to follow the alkaline diet and you will lose weight and will feel healthier sooner.

6. Break the Laziness

In the previous chapters, it was discussed over and over again how the alkaline meals can boost the energy of a person. So make the most of that energy and use it for the betterment of your health and body. Just because you are already on an alkaline diet doesn't mean that you can stop moving around. If you don't know what kind of activity to do, refer to number 2.

7. Avoid Constipation

Even with alkaline diet, you may encounter moments when it's hard to eliminate body waste. When this problem occurs, eat lots of foods rich in fiber (see chapter 1). And don't forget to drink lots of alkaline water.

8. Make Huge Amounts of Salads (Good for 3 days)

It isn't often that a person finds enough time to do everything in a day. You may sometimes feel like you barely have enough time to breathe. When this happens, it may be tempting to compromise and simply fall into the old habit of taking whatever food is available. In order to be consistent in following your alkaline diet, set a day where you can make a big bowl of salad which can last for at least three days. So when you have to deal with emergency cases and have no time to prepare or buy alkaline meals, you can simply pack some salad in your meal box and you're good to go.

Now, you already have learned the facts about alkaline diet. You also found ways to achieve a healthier way of living life and the safest way of losing weight. There is no shortcut to success. But when you apply everything that you have learned from this book, you will eventually reach the success like many others who have already tried this diet.

So go ahead, start making those alkaline recipes, and enjoy   a   healthy   fit   body.

A FINAL WORD

An alkaline diet is not only recommended to shed those extra pounds but is also and more importantly a great means of regaining lost health and leading a longer and more diseases free life. This diet is especially recommended to those who feel tired most of the time. Stress and a low energy level can both be done away with a diet that is acid alkaline.

Those who suffer from frequent viral fevers or those who have a nasal congestion most of the time can lead healthier lives if they have a diet that is acid alkaline. Weak nails, dryness, headaches, muscle pain, hives, joint pains, and many more such diseases find their answer in an alkaline ash diet.

Please Leave a Review

Finally, if you enjoyed this book, please take the time to share your thoughts and post a review on Amazon. It would be greatly appreciated.

That review and feedback will help me improve the content in my books – and make each and every one more relevant and helpful to you.

Thank you again and good luck!

J.C. Collins